Tap
Out
Emotional
Pain

Use This Emotional Freedom
Technique to Improve
Your Health and Wellness

RON KNESS

Contents

Disclaimer

This publication is for informational purposes only and is not intended as medical advice. Medical advice should always be obtained from a qualified medical professional for any health conditions or symptoms associated with them.

Every possible effort has been made in preparing and researching this material. We make no warranties with respect to the accuracy, applicability of its contents or any omissions.

See your healthcare professional before starting any diet or exercise program!

Introduction

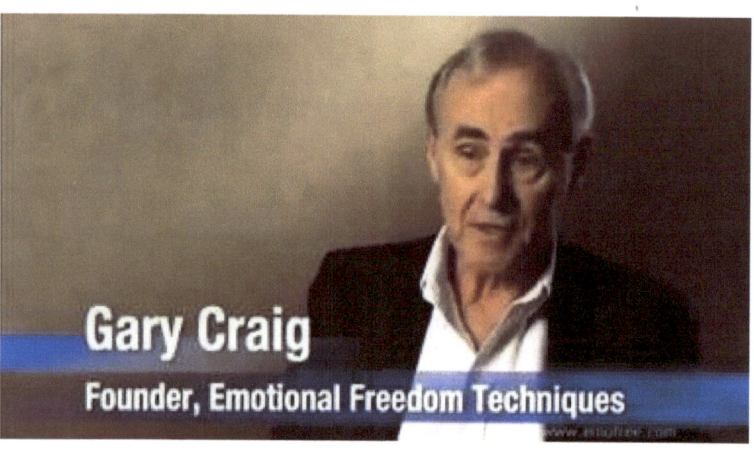

Gary Craig
Founder, Emotional Freedom Techniques

Brief History of EFT Development

Gary Craig (born April 13, 1940) is a Stanford engineering graduate and the founder and creator of EFT, which has been developed and added to since 1995. His daughter, Tina Craig, has worked with him over many years and helped in perfecting and making refinements to the teaching of the technique.

Gary is not a licensed therapist or psychologist but an ordained minister with the Universal Church of God in Southern California--a non-denominational church that embraces all religions. He is also a Certified Master Practitioner in NLP (Neuro Linguistic Programming). He has always been very interested in personal development and improvement. He states that the highest levels of healing can be achieved with the tool of EFT, the core of which he learned from Dr. Roger Callahan. He is self-taught (as is his daughter), basing his work on a recognition that quality of thought is mirrored in quality of life.

Unresolved Emotional Issues Are at the Heart of Every Malady

The Chinese discovered a system of invisible energy channels flowing through the body around 5000 years ago. These channels are known as meridians, and dominate most healing disciplines in the East. This system is the basis for acupuncture and acupressure, and also other healing practices. It is also the basis for EFT (Emotional Freedom Techniques).

With television, you do not see the electrical energy flowing through the wires connected to your TV set, but its presence is evident by the effects produced--you get sound and picture. Likewise, the body's energy systems are not seen by the eyes, however, their effects are felt and can be adjusted and aligned by tapping near the meridian endpoints. Striking changes can occur in physical, emotional, motivational and performance health and ability.

Emotional Freedom Techniques (also known as EFT or sometimes simply called Tapping) is a technique that uses a sort of acupressure to tap on various acupuncture points and follows along the body's meridians or invisible energy channels. It works with psychological and emotional issues which are often overlooked in traditional success-oriented and healing methods. Optimal diet and a pristine lifestyle alone do not assure you will have ideal health and have the energy and emotional mindset to achieve all your goals.

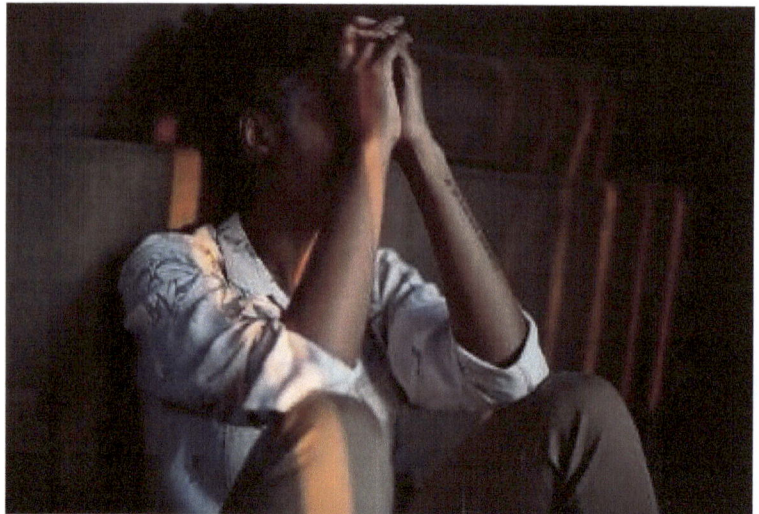

Emotional issues should be targeted for results that last the longest and are the most powerful, although there are cases involving physical symptoms which respond well to EFT which bypass the emotional involvement, and give relief when EFT is applied directly to the physical symptom.

EFT is a tool that has been shown to give impressive results in virtually all areas of human desire whether it be issues involving emotional, physical, or performance issues.

What is the Premise of EFT?

The premise of EFT is that there are always emotional issues getting in the way of achieving your goals, no matter if they are in the area of health or pain (physical issues), or emotional blocks to achieving success. It has long been known that emotional stresses or subconscious resistance can get in the way of the body's natural healing processes and can prevent you from moving forward with your goals.

There is another premise that EFT holds: As you get to clearing more and more unresolved emotional issues that can be standing in the way (and realistically, we all have some emotional issues that are limiting us from complete freedom and happiness), the greater the peace and freedom you can achieve. Imagine vigorous good health, thriving, healthy relationships, and freedom from limiting beliefs with the resulting exceptional performance heights and achievements.

EFT is fluid and ongoing and can wipe out old traumas, whether they be physical or emotional. It is a process that is expansive and welcoming of challenges.

Can EFT Work without Delving into Underlying Emotional Issues?

The mechanism of EFT can be stated very simply in one sentence, which is called The Discovery Statement: "The cause of all negative emotions is a disruption in the body's energy system."

Conventional psychotherapy presumes a connection between negative emotions and some past traumatic experience that those emotions are caused by traumatic past memories. EFT treatment respects the memory but does not require the client to relive painful past events. Instead, EFT simply addresses the disruption of the body's energy system.

Many people think that it is necessary to delve deeply into memory details of their past traumas for EFT to help them. The tapping process does not require any of that.

Although the memories may contribute to undesirable emotions, this has nothing to do with their cause, and it is unnecessary, and possibly even damaging, to dwell on or dredge up these painful memories.

Using EFT involves very little, if any, emotional suffering. Just a brief recall of the problem, which can involve some discomfort, but nothing beyond that. Any prolonged emotional discomfort would indicate it is not being done correctly.

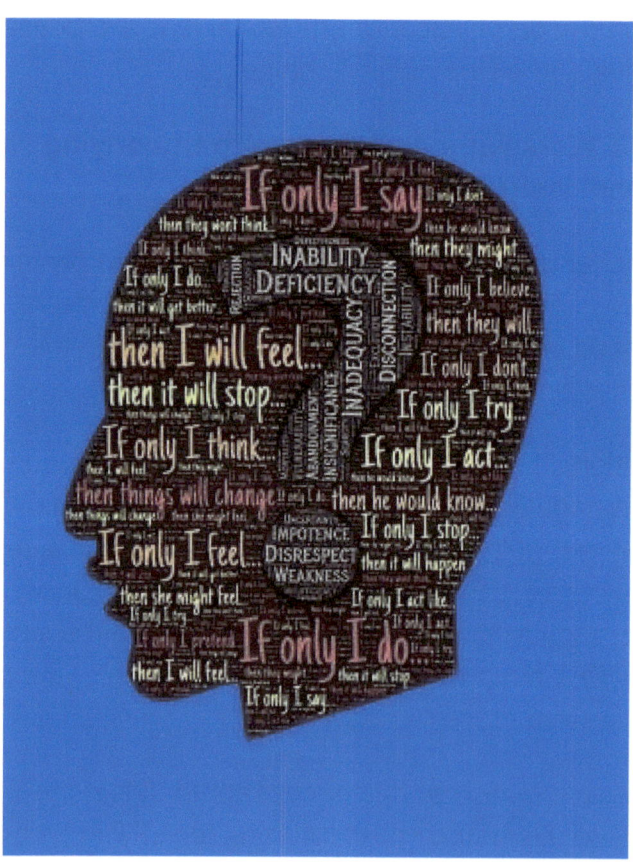

If the energy flow system in the body becomes imbalanced, there is a disruption of the flow which can result in a negative emotion being generated. During the application of EFT

Tapping, energy is re-routed to its normal and proper channels and the negative emotion fades away. It is simple and very effective, though it may be hard to believe that such a simple process can work so well.

As with the energy systems established with acupuncture and acupressure points, you are tapping into the same system, but literally tapping with your fingertips below the skin's surface, along the same meridian channels. As you are doing this, you are mentally focused on some emotional issue or stress. This causes the body's alarm system to get activated, but tapping at the same time brings on the signal for relaxation, thus teaching the body to give a different response to the stressor. The sessions give not only emotional relief and diminished physical symptoms, but also some impressive cognitive shifts.

What Makes Tapping So Effective?

How Do the Tapping Points Correspond with EFT?

The EFT tapping points correspond to acupuncture points in the body's meridians that are major channels. There are three fundamental energy channels within our fingertips that come together (Central, Right Main, and Left Main Channels). In Taoist Chi Gung Theory, these three channels form before we are born, while in the womb. From these, other meridians branch out within the body.

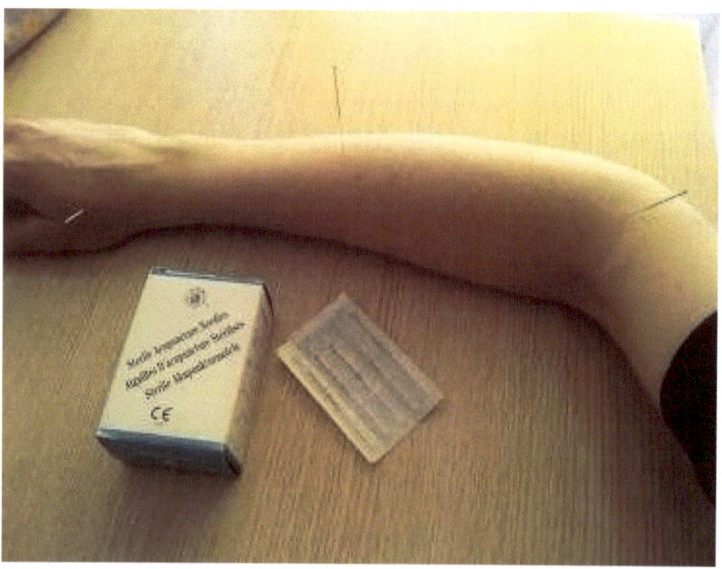

Lymphatic congestion builds up at the right EFT sore spot and the karate chop point of the right hand. This sore spot point is located on each side of the thymus gland, about 3 inches to the left or right. Through the left hand karate chop point and the left EFT sore spot flow the Central and Left Main Channels.

By What Mechanism Does EFT Work at an Emotional Level?

Think of the meridians as energy highways, carrying information to the various body destinations. Massive amounts of energy are absorbed by the body every day, everywhere we go, as we take in data from our experiences. We also receive internal information at a subconscious level, of biochemical activity going on at the tissue and cellular levels, such as basal temperature, pH, and sugar balances.

How Can EFT Help to Process All That Information?

When we tap using the EFT process, our attention is focused inward. Information that was hidden from conscious awareness but which is associated with our tapping issue, comes to the surface. Any negative feelings that arise give us clues to energy disruptions that have taken place and that are linked to the information that is surfacing.

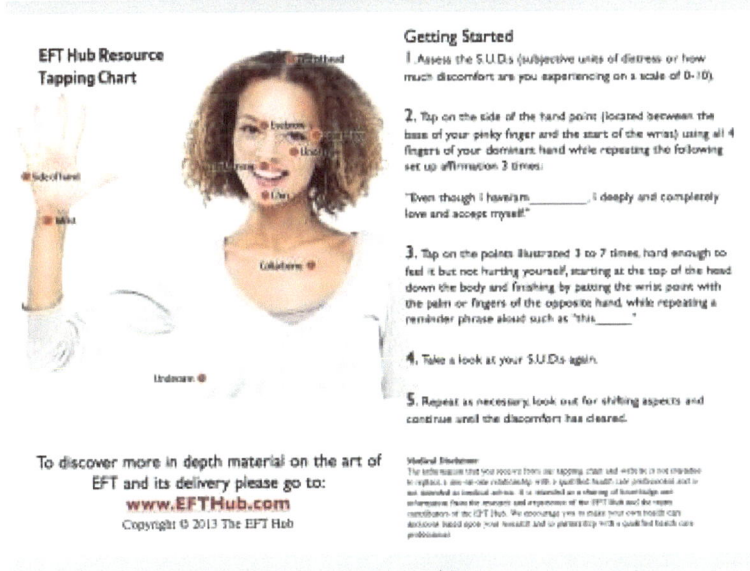

Tapping allows the release of negative emotions. This unblocks the energy before the corresponding physical body parts get bogged down with stagnant energy and start to express disease. Various traumas caused by intense events in our lives carry with them strong negative emotions. Often we are overwhelmed with the emotions and are not able to fully process and release them.

So many of us have developed unhealthy coping mechanisms for these strong negative emotions that have not been fully processed. We tend to pretend they don't exist, stuff them or stay distracted to avoid handling them.

Without acknowledgement, these emotions are never properly released; they stay submerged and operate unconsciously. They cause continuous short-circuiting of the energy meridians whenever something triggers a traumatic memory and brings it into awareness, causing it to surface. Our energy system keeps trying to clear the disconnect as negative emotions keep trying to be released.

How Are Trauma-Induced Energy Disruptions Cleared Through EFT?

Any time we are caught up in an overwhelming situation, a barrage of intense emotions, thoughts, and physical sensations overtake us in an energy blast that floods through our systems. Our meridians and the points along the way attempt to contain and move the excess energy along.

On occasion, though, such an experience generates an overload of the energy system. The system can crash just the same way a computer can crash when there's an information overload or a power surge.

The tapping techniques of EFT help to alleviate much of the burden caused by the excess trapped energy that is contained in the memory of the traumatic event.

As you go through the tapping procedure, you give attention to the wide range of emotions that may surface, and acknowledge each until gradually each one is released. Thus the excess energy gets cleared and balance gets restored to the system.

It may help to think of energy disruption in the meridian system like a river that has multiple tributaries. A small amount of debris floating in the water probably won't interfere too much with the flow. The river is able to carry it off. But if there is a continuous influx of debris or a very massive amount dumped in suddenly as with a trauma, the current gets bogged down and over time, stagnates.

Once the debris settles, it can completely block the flow of the river, causing water to get backed up in some places, equivalent to an excess of energy or depriving some areas of water completely, equivalent to an energy deficit. This is like constant stress in the body, building up over time, or being hit with a big emotional trauma that causes an energy irregularity.

If the energy blockage is severe enough, a reversal of energy may occur. You may feel so drained of energy that you can hardly do anything.

How Can EFT Unblock Emotions?

In EFT, we start with what is called a set-up statement. In the setup statement, you are acknowledging that a problem exists and you are stating that it is okay that you have that problem. With the setup statement, you are allowing the emotion to be as it is, without resistance and without self-rejection. As you focus in with complete acceptance and assign an intensity rating to the problem, you are bringing the emotion right into the present.

Here the emotion is safe to be felt and expressed because a distinction is made: the problem may be unacceptable, but that does not make ourselves unacceptable. We are completely accepting of ourselves, just as we are. As we focus on the issue and the emotion that accompanies it, an activation of the underlying energy disruption takes place. As this is happening, the timing of the tapping is in sync with the energy disruption. This pushes the energy through, to restore the correct and natural flow.

As we tap, we can observe the tapping issue decrease in intensity or change. We see ourselves as the observer. It becomes easier to release the emotion as we recognize that we are not under the emotion's control.

How effective is EFT with Painful Trauma?

Wherever there are emotions, there is usually strong energy. The charge of that energy can be either positive or negative. When working with EFT, we do not need to be immersed in the strong charge of the pain that may as yet be unreleased.

The intensity of the emotion that accompanies the issue should first be lessened before commencing in a step-by-step manner with other emotions, gradually going deeper, as with peeling an onion. It is not recommended to forge right into the heaviest part of the emotion when attempting to release the charge.

The sequence is to start on the outermost area of emotion and proceed slowly, layer by layer. Be advised, there may be occasions when there is an unexpected plunge into the heart of a deep trauma, bringing up sudden, intense emotions.

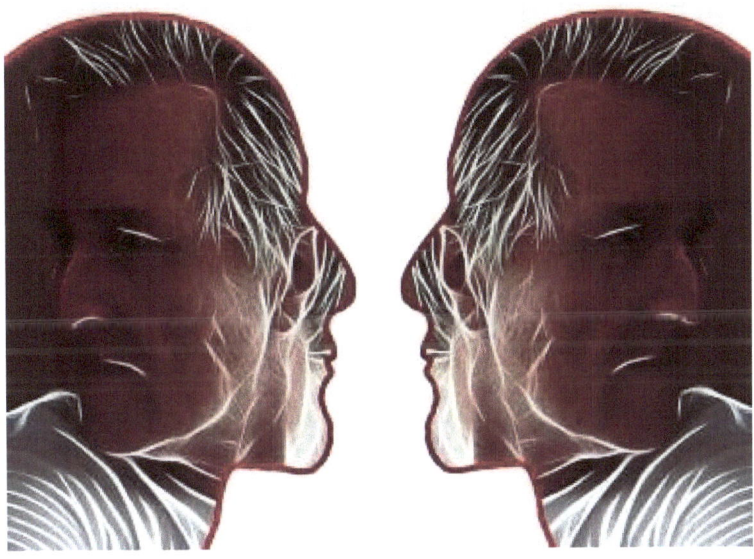

Such new memories uncovered may take us totally off guard, especially if they have been forgotten or we assumed they were previously resolved. At times, this situation can happen with such rapidity that we are not able to advance into it slowly. If this should happen, the remedy is to tap quickly and continuously through all the points until that emotional energy dissipates and gets released.

The Science and Research Behind EFT Tapping

The Fight-or-Flight Response

Our bodies were designed to prepare us to be ready for dangerous threats, an evolutionary trait that goes back to the cave man being chased by a saber-toothed cat misleadingly known as a saber-toothed tiger. The body prepares to either stay and fight, or flee the danger. Heart rate, blood pressure and blood sugar levels rise so that you have the energy needed to fight or run. Your muscles get tense, and adrenaline floods your system for energy.

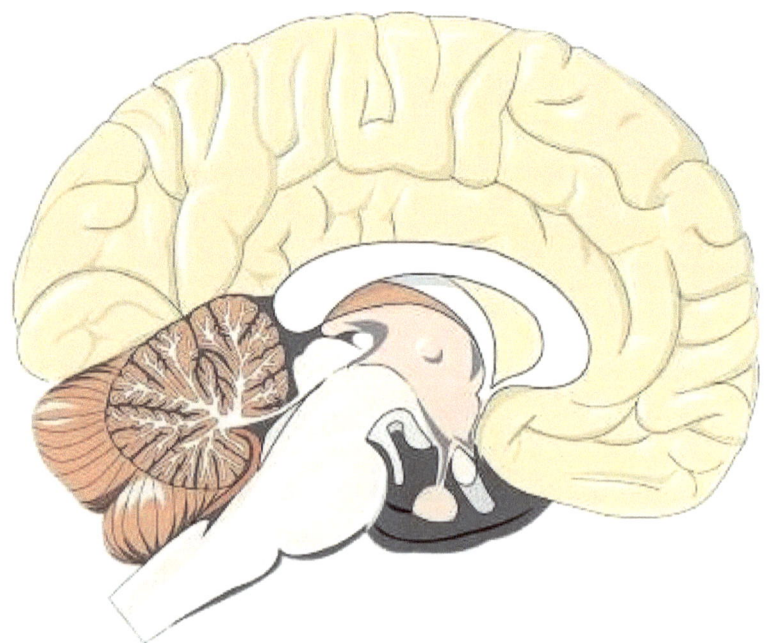

The response to stress like that was very real, but in more recent times, that fight-or-flight response is overkill for most of our stresses, yet it still gets activated, even if the stress is internal. Adrenaline still pumps and heart rate quickens. A past trauma, negative memory or conditioned childhood response can trigger the same body reactions. Tapping short-circuits the fight-or-flight response, allowing a different response from the brain and body.

The Role of the Brain's Amygdala

Within the brain is an almond-shaped body called the amygdala, part of the limbic system (midbrain), which is where emotions, long-term memory, and negative experiences reside. According to scientific research, the amygdala initiates the stress response by alerting the brain to ready the body in preparation for the fight-or-flight mechanism.

What Happens When EFT Calms the Body's Alarm System?

When we tap on the meridian endpoints, this creates a calming response throughout the body by deactivating the amygdala's warning alarm and resetting the system.

A hormone called cortisol floods the system when the stress response is activated. Tapping helps to reduce the levels of cortisol so that the body can initiate repair, renewal and normalizing functions.

It is not fully understood why tapping on the meridian end points resets the amygdala's alarm, but a calming response is sent to the body. The amygdala gets a message that all is well, the organism is safe, and it shuts down its alarm.

What Is the Mechanism That Makes Tapping Work?

As previously stated, the body functions using electro-chemical energy. The acupuncture meridians are like channels to conduct energy currents. Anytime the circuit gets disrupted, it causes a physical or emotional discomfort, or both.

When the energy flow in the body gets disrupted, certain areas of the body may get too little, while others get an excess. Physically tapping with fingertips on the facial and body acupuncture points resets and re-balances the energy so that it can once again flow freely and properly as it is meant to do. Many practitioners have come to understand that there is a mind-body link affecting emotions, stress, and illness.

Research Defeats Skepticism

EFT has as its basis, a root in the ancient wisdom, and modern healing practitioners like doctors and psychologists have viewed it with a healthy dose of skepticism. However, there is a mounting pile of anecdotal evidence that it works, from people who have used it with great success.

Evidence is accumulating with undeniable research indicating real breakthroughs produced by EFT in conditions which often were not helped by conventional medicine or psychotherapy. Studies coming out of the prestigious Harvard Medical School during the past ten years are lending credence to the claims. Stress and the fear response, controlled by the brain's amygdala, can be dampened when meridian point stimulation is applied through the use of acupuncture, acupressure, and EFT tapping.

Admittedly, the studies were based on results using acupuncture and needles; however, a double-blind follow-up indicated that pressure stimulation of the meridian points, (as in tapping) also gave similar outcomes.

Impressive Statistics from the Research of Dr. Church

Additionally, Dr. Dawson Church and a team of his conducted a randomized controlled trial. They measured cortisol levels on 83 test subjects. Cortisol, again, is that hormone that the body produces whenever it is exposed to a stressful event. Average cortisol reduction levels dropped to 24%, and as much as almost 50% in some participants. Comparatively, no significant reduction of cortisol was observed in subjects receiving an entire hour of traditional talk therapy.

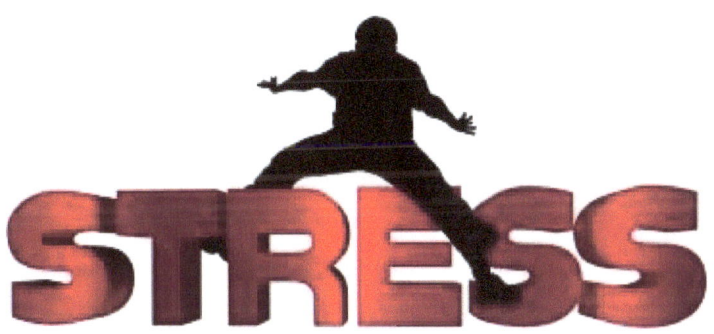

What EFT Has Done for PTSD Sufferers

Dr. Church is responsible for teaching the tapping method to post-traumatic stress disorder (PTSD) sufferers who are war veterans, with a program called The Stress Project.

Extremely impressive results are showing up with averages of a 63% drop in PTSD symptoms after six rounds of tapping. Such results are turning around the skeptic beliefs of the scientific community.

The war veterans suffering from PTSD have responded particularly well to EFT treatment. PTSD has been difficult to treat. Antidepressant and antipsychotic drugs work about as effectively as placebos, according to studies.

Operation: Emotional Freedom is a documentary film directed by Eric Huurre, which follows veterans and their families as they go through some very intensive EFT therapy conducted by Gary Craig and other EFT practitioners. These veterans were all suffering from PTSD, anxiety and depression due to their combat experiences. Some were suicidal. Following the EFT treatment, the results were quite impressive. Each described renewed feelings of peacefulness and hope. They were conquering their emotional traumas of combat.

The documentary examines health care available currently for PTSD-diagnosed war veterans, and looks at the drug approach being offered as treatment for the emotional issues these veterans are experiencing. It points up the myths and misconceptions of this approach to treatment. Drugs are not meeting the challenge as pharmaceutical companies had originally claimed.

How You Get Physical Relief Though the Emotional Door

All Disease Has One Root Cause

The Discovery Statement makes the assertion that "The cause of ALL negative emotions is a disruption in the body's energy system." This is all inclusive--it includes all forms of anxiety and phobias, all fears, anger, PTSD, grief, depression, all memories that bring back traumatic events, all types of worry, guilt, and all limiting beliefs having to do with any performance issues, either in business, the performing arts, sports, or any other artistic endeavors. That comprehensive statement encompasses virtually every emotion we can experience that is restrictive or limiting in any way. What it means is that EVERY negative emotion has but one root cause = an electrical misalignment or short-circuiting of the energy that can be rebooted and normalized by the same simple method.

The Simplified Solution

Any trauma, then, or fear, guilt, grief or even a hockey player's performance slump is originating out of the same root cause. Therefore, the same method, in general terms, will work for all these issues. This becomes a relief for mental health professionals when they embrace the idea since it simplifies their work. With so many emotional crises clients can have, mental health professionals needed to be constantly offering up numerous explanations and therapies to help their clients, often with less than encouraging results.

Understanding that there is really only one cause makes their work easier and more effective.

Emotional Issues Directly Affect the Chemistry of the Body

It has long been acknowledged by the medical profession that our body chemistry can be strongly affected by our emotions. All sorts of maladies and diseases can erupt from this chain of events, from disorders resulting from an impaired immune system, to addictions, circulatory problems, inflammation, cancer, or headaches and rashes.

Apply the simple Tapping process to resolve issues that have an emotional component, such as fear, anger, guilt, emotional trauma, etc., and it is quite common for physical ailments to be resolved right along with the emotional afflictions. It is also possible sometimes to see physical ailments subside with simple tapping on the meridian system, not involving the EFT process in any emotional components. This suggests that an energetic factor was contributing to the physical affliction, and symptoms could be alleviated simply by meridian re-balancing.

How to Do EFT Tapping

Start by Focusing on Some Negative Emotion

There are some basic principles to understand. To start, you will focus on a negative emotion that is a problem for you. It can be a bad memory you cannot seem to shake, or some anxiety or fear or any unresolved issue you are trying to get control over. As you are keeping this issue in mind, you will use your fingertips to give 5-7 taps on each of 12 meridian points of the body. To get to a state of balance, and thus, restore the body's natural energy, you focus on accepting and resolving the negative issue as you tap.

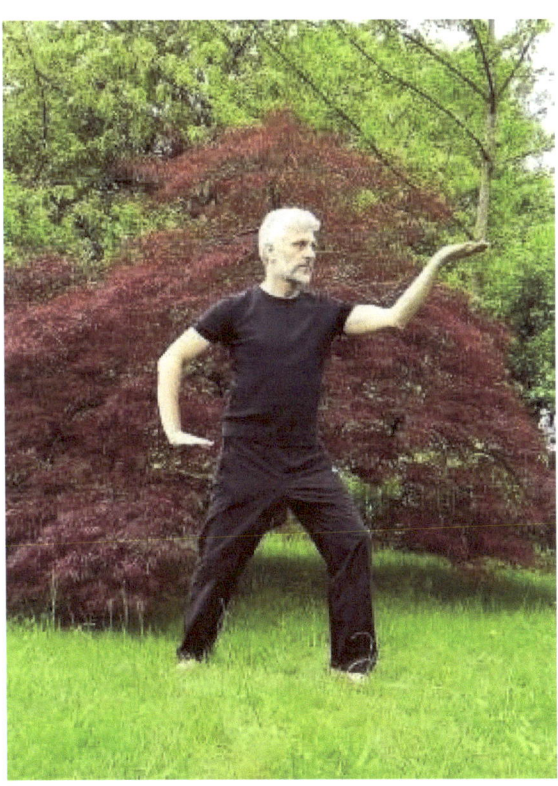

Tap into Your Meridian Channels

It is an amazing discovery which emerged out of traditional Chinese medicine, that energy, called chi, travels along the meridian channels, and it is possible to tap into and re-balance this energy at any point along the way. The Chinese uncovered 100 acupuncture points that, when stimulated with thin needles, restored balance of the life force energy and effected healing of the body.

The Advantages of Tapping versus Acupuncture

Tapping is very similar to acupuncture, except there are no needles involved, so it is painless and while mastering acupuncture takes years of study and practice, EFT is very simple and quick to learn by virtually anyone. There is no need to memorize the hundreds of meridian points located throughout the body. You can work on yourself anytime, just about anywhere that you happen to be. It takes less time to perform than acupuncture and is certainly less expensive. And most astonishingly--it can be applied towards virtually any emotional issues or challenges you face in your life. The power to heal yourself or improve and motivate yourself is in your own hands; you have complete control.

The Tapping Sequence

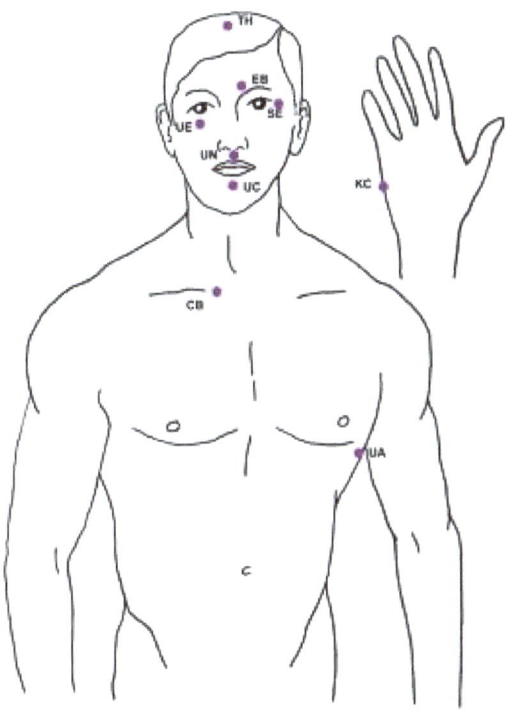

To start with the basics, here are the nine points, in the correct order that you will be tapping on, with some brief explanations. Go to http://eft.mercola.com/ to see photos of the exact tapping points and how to place your hands. You can also watch a short video demonstration on this site.

1. Top of the Head. Start with the top of the head. You are using both hands, backs of fingers facing each other, at the center of the skull.

2. Eyebrow. Just above the nose but at the beginning of the eyebrows.

3. Side of the eyes. On the bone right at the outside corner of the eyes.

4. Directly under the eyes.

5. Under the center of the nose, just above the upper lip.

6. Chin. Halfway between the lower lip and the actual edge of the chin bone.

7. Collar Bone. Find the notch at the top of the sternum, where a man's tie knot falls. From the bottom of this notch, go down about one inch and one inch to the left or right. This is not technically the collar bone but it is referred to as such for simplicity.

8. Under the arm. About four inches below the armpit on the side of the body.

9. Wrists. On the inside of both wrists, each wrist tapping on the other.

Affirmations

Why Should You Do Affirmations?

Affirmations are a way to pamper yourself, to be kind to yourself and, in a sense, soothe and caress your mind. It can be viewed that every thought and sentence you say to yourself is a sort of affirmation. Of course, these can be either negative or positive. And when you do intentional and very specific affirmations, you are greatly enhancing the effectiveness of EFT.

How do you start? First think up a positive statement that lifts your spirits instead of bringing you down or beating yourself up. These statements affirm something you wish to do or make; something that affirms a goal you want to achieve.

Any positive self-statement that you start with initiates the process. If the statement feels false to you at the beginning, that's okay--just keep repeating it to yourself many times during the day. You are reprogramming your subconscious mind, and soon it will begin to accept the statements as true, because the subconscious mind does not distinguish about what is really true or not--it simply accepts what it is hearing, especially if it hears it over and over again.

When Should Affirmations Be Done?

These affirmations should be repeated upon arising in the morning, and just before you go to sleep at night. It is at this time that it is most important.

As you tap right before you go to sleep and repeat your affirmations, your subconscious mind has the full sleep-time to process the affirmations and prepare to create those results for you in your life. You can also get into the habit of saying them every time you make a trip to the bathroom.

If prayer is comforting to you, you can incorporate your prayers into your EFT self-talk and that, too, will increase the effectiveness along with your affirmations. The sooner you get into the habit of nightly tapping and affirmations, the greater the benefit and the sooner the process will begin working for you.

Working with a Mirror

A very effective and inexpensive technique is to look into a mirror as you tap. Looking deeply into your own eyes seems to enhance the connection with your own subconscious mind. Instead of the energy you are stimulating going off into space, the mirror seems to be reflecting your energy back to you. This is a very simple technique but can be very powerful in its effect.

Is Your Mind Sending You Negative Messages?

As you peer into your mirror and commence doing your affirmations, tap on all the EFT points. Stay focused and alert to what you may hear internally. Initially, no messages may come through. If any negative self-talk comes up, this can be thwarting progress. If you tend to beat yourself up, you may not be used to hearing gentle and loving thoughts. Keep listening and you will learn self-trust and confidence as you also start feeling better about yourself.

Some of us beat ourselves up for every little mistake, even if it is quite small and insignificant. You may not fall into this category, but everyone can use a daily dose of self-forgiveness, and your mirror is a great tool here, too.

Here is a very powerful technique: Get in front of your mirror. Look directly into your own eyes and say, "Even though I got angry or impatient . . . or I was unsuccessful in my efforts" (or whatever the issue may be that you need to forgive yourself for), then say, "I forgive you. You were doing the best you could."

Continue with, "I forgive you for holding on to these patterns so long. I forgive you for not loving yourself." You are looking into your own eyes as you say the word, "you." If there is a negative thought, be sure to acknowledge it but not give it too much importance. If the negative thought arises, use EFT to counteract it so that a positive opposite is generated. When you try this, you will see how powerful a technique this really is.

5 Points to Keep in Mind as You Practice EFT

Focusing In on the Issue

Specificity is very important, especially with the language that is used. You will need to be very focused and concentrating on the issue that is being addressed. It is common, if the subject is an emotionally painful one, to want to disconnect from the painful feelings. You may find yourself getting distracted, pulled away by other thoughts, or otherwise disengaged. It is important to continue to stay connected.

When Reframing Occurs

Even in one round of tapping, there will be energy movement and it is vital to pay close attention as a shift in the energy occurs. Any time you see the issue from a new perspective, a cognitive shift has occurred and a reframing of the issue will emerge. It can creep up unexpectedly with new insight. An energy shift such as this can present a valuable association not seen before. This can broaden new avenues for healing to take place. After such a shift, there is often a release of self-blame and guilt. You may experience a renewed feeling of hopefulness, or simply a feeling of relief that had been absent previously.

The Importance of Body Hydration

The importance of good hydration cannot be overemphasized, both for the client and the practitioner. Water is a strong conductor of electricity.

Electrical energy flows continuously through the body and brain, through positively and negatively charged ions (atoms that have one or more electrons removed or added, thus giving them an electrical charge). The practice of EFT Tapping accesses this electrically-charged energy, and that is why it is essential to maintain proper hydration. It is recommended to consume approximately one quart per day of pure water per each fifty pounds of body weight.

How is Healing Accomplished?

Gary Craig reminds us that the healing takes place through the practitioner when the client is open to receive that healing; it is not healing by the practitioner that occurs. Just as all hypnosis is really self-hypnosis, only the client himself does the healing and any practitioner who claims to be the healer can actually interfere with the process. The facilitator can only witness the activity and feel humble to have played a part in helping the client to create his or her own healing development.

Your Responsibility

You have a responsibility to take care of yourself, only doing what feels right. If you are working with a trained practitioner, make sure you are not going into issues that are causing emotional distress or that feel threatening.

Final Thoughts

Just about any skill that you want to learn to do takes regular practice. We understand that and don't question it. For our emotional health, it's the same way. Even small practices that are done routinely over a long period of time add up and give us a good outcome--the outcome we are hoping for.

What does it mean to get into the routine of a practice? It means doing that routine on a regular basis, ideally at the same time every day, and sticking to it, no matter what the resistance or distractions or whatever else comes up to get us off track. We make the commitment because we get the results we desire. It is a way of fighting against complacency, against habitual old and outdated emotions, attitudes and beliefs, and old behaviors that do not serve us in the long run.

There are lots of practices you can find to do that are of great benefit and that will improve your life. Meditation is one, of course, but one of the best, and sadly, probably passed over too frequently, is getting into a Tapping practice, a regular routine of tapping. Anytime you perform a round of tapping will be of benefit, but it is best if you use tapping on a consistent basis. Unfortunately, like so many things that are good for us, when we are not in the habit of doing them, when an emergency occurs and the practice is needed the most, we forget about using it. We just don't think of it.

Of course it's a good idea to tap whenever a situation arises, but it is even better to set your intention and make it something you do regularly.

A daily practice is best, and more frequently when you are ill. You decide what time of day is most convenient for you. Some people prefer early in the morning; for others, in the evening or just before bed works best. You also decide how long the duration should be for you. It is best to choose a time and duration that will be easy to keep up with on a continual basis, so you can succeed with your intention.

A good plan is to set up a chart showing the days of the week that you are committed to your practice. Again, daily is best for the most progress, but choose whatever is realistic for you. Check off each session after completing it. If you fail to do this, you can end up skipping several days before you even realize you've fallen off the program. Seeing those empty boxes not checked off will serve as your reminder to stay with it.

There can still be resistance, even if you have your intention set, you love the idea, and you are fully aware of the benefits. Even the most ardent tappers still succumb to occasional missed sessions because they didn't have the time or forgot or couldn't think of what to tap on. It is crucial when this happens not to go beating yourself up!

Understand that the part that has failed to keep up with the practice is the part that needs the most love and support. Some part of you may be harboring feelings of unworthiness or wanting to punish yourself by not doing the nurturing thing. Tapping is a way to give self-love. By tapping, we are giving care and nurturing to ourselves, tending to our emotional health and well-being, and honoring ourselves. At these times, instead of judging yourself, bring the message of love.

What is it we all want? To feel loved and accepted, to know we are loving and accepting individuals. We all seek happiness, fulfillment and peace. By committing to a regular practice of tapping, you will bring to yourself that continuous stream of acceptance and love. The deep, profoundly transformative healing that your soul yearns for will be yours.

References

http://www.emofree.com/eft-tutorial/tapping-basics/what-is-eft.html

http://eft.mercola.com/

http://www.goodvibrationsenergymedicine.com/HOME/Sessions-By-Modality/Energy-Meridian-Tapping-Techniques-TFT-and-EFT

http://www.thetappingsolution.com/

http://www.tapintoyourcenter.com/services/mindset-eft

http://articles.mercola.com/sites/articles/archive/2013/12/26/emotional-freedom-technique.aspx

http://www.healing-with-eft.com/how-does-eft-work.html

http://www.eftuniverse.com/index.php?option=com_content&view=article&id=3753:the-qproper-wordsq-for-the-eft-set-up-statement&catid=33:articles-a-ideas&Itemid=3147

Other Relevant Health Books by This Author

If you would like to read more about Senior Health and Fitness, here is a list of the <u>titles, CreateSpace links and descriptions:</u>

<u>https://www.createspace.com/5457441</u>

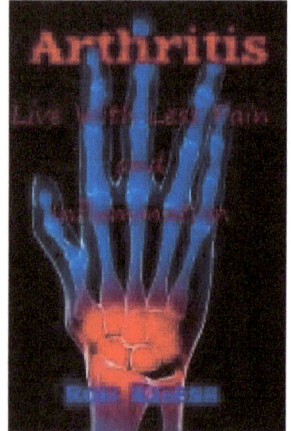

<u>Arthritis - Live with Less Pain and Inflammation</u>

You learn things like:
• Simple and effective information that will help you manage the pain and inflammation that comes along with arthritis, so that you can live an active, full life without debilitating pain.
• The different types of arthritis, their symptoms and how to alleviate their painful side effects.
• The pros and cons of over-the-counter arthritis medications, plus simple tips that will help you know how to choose the right supplements.
• Free, yet effective ways to get relief from arthritis pain and inflammation, so you don't have to suffer anymore.
the effects arthritis can have significant impact on your physical and mental well-being, but this books shows you how to overcome its painful symptoms and live life relatively pain free.

https://www.createspace.com/5519874

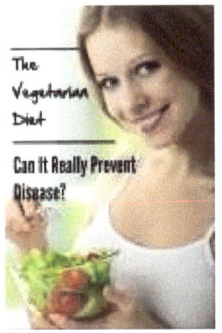

The Vegetarian Diet – Can It Really Prevent Disease?

Is a vegetarian diet right for you? Multiple studies have shown over and over that a vegetarian diet goes along way in preventing certain chronic diseases, such as:

• Heart Disease
• Cancer
• Diverticulitis
• Type 2 Diabetes
• Hypertension
• Obesity
• Kidney Failure

https://www.createspace.com/5714434

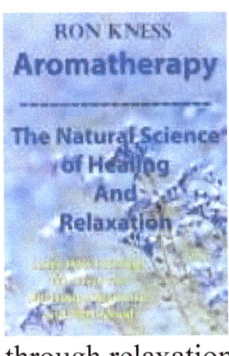

Aromatherapy - The Science of Healing and Relaxation: Learn How Essential Oils Elicit The Relaxation Response And Alter Mood

In my book, we reveal the natural holistic methods you can use to heal the body from certain medical issues and to relive stress through relaxation. In particular we talk about:

• Aromatherapy - what it is and how it works
• Essential Oils – how the effects of certain aromas differs from others
• Recipes – how to make your own essential oil combinations

Learn how to reap the benefits of using essential oils as part of your aromatherapy.

https://www.createspace.com/6651022

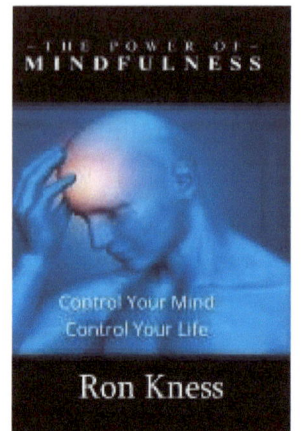

The Power of Mindfulness

If there is one ability you could learn that would make every single aspect of your life better, what would it be?

Undoubtedly, it would be the ability to control your emotions and the way you think.

This might sound like a surprising claim, but the ability to control your emotions and the way you respond to a situation is not only the secret to happiness, but the secret to being able to get whatever you want from life.

Why? Because it's our interpretation of events more than the events themselves that dictate our happiness, mood and performance. Not only that but our emotions, and the neurotransmitters that control them, are what alter our ability to focus, to remember information and to be creative.

Here's what you'll discover inside...
 - Exactly what mindfulness is and how to start using it in daily life...

- The simple mindfulness exercises you can start using today to begin getting more control over your mind than you've ever had before...

- An overview of CBT, or cognitive behavior therapy, and why it's incredibly powerful...

- How to use CBT in real world situations to overcome fear and anxiety in your daily life...

- How to use mindfulness to improve your success with the opposite sex and dating...

- What causes stress in your life and how to overcome it by changing your thoughts...

- Why the age old fight or flight response can actually be hurting you more than helping you in today's modern life...

- You may have "hidden powers" and not even realize it… discover how to tap into your hidden powers using mindfulness...

- The power of visualization and how to use it in your life to get more of what you want...

- How to become socially fearless with hypothesis testing...

- The Law of Attraction and how to use it for a life of abundance...

- Plus, a whole lot more...

This is the most complete guide to harnessing the power of mindfulness that you'll ever find…

In short, this book is going to show you how to simply get some peace and quiet by calming your mind and taking a time out. Read on and get ready to change your life…

About the Author

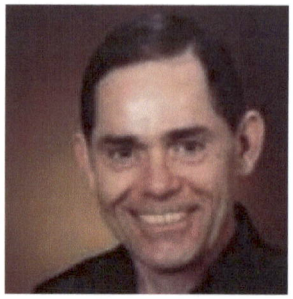

I grew up in Central Minnesota, where my parents owned and operated a fishing resort. Once out of high school I tried a couple of semesters of college, only to quit halfway through the Spring term; I decided at that time that college wasn't for me.

Then I decided to follow my father's previous occupation as an auto mechanic. I graduated from a two-year of vocational training course and worked as a mechanic for five years. While in vocational training, I decided to join the National Guard where I eventually ended up working full-time for 32 years.

So how does all of this relate to writing? In one of my leadership schools, the instructor, who was an English teacher at a juvenile detention center, presented writing to me in a whole new way - a way that started to develop my interest in working with words.

I eventually went back to college on the GI Bill while I was working and earned my Bachelor's degree in Business Administration. Taking a class or two per semester at night and on weekends took me seven years to complete my degree.

Fast forward about 40 years and I now have published over 75 books on Amazon for Kindle, CreateSpace and other publishing platforms.

Besides my own writing, I also ghostwrite ebooks, reports, articles, blogs and do Kindle conversions for clients on a variety of topics.

Today my wife and I are retired from our careers and live in Gold Canyon, AZ. I now write as a retirement business where you'll find me happily sitting in my office typing away on my laptop as I work on my next book or ghostwriting project . . . that is if we are not traveling on a cruise ship - our new-found mode of travel.